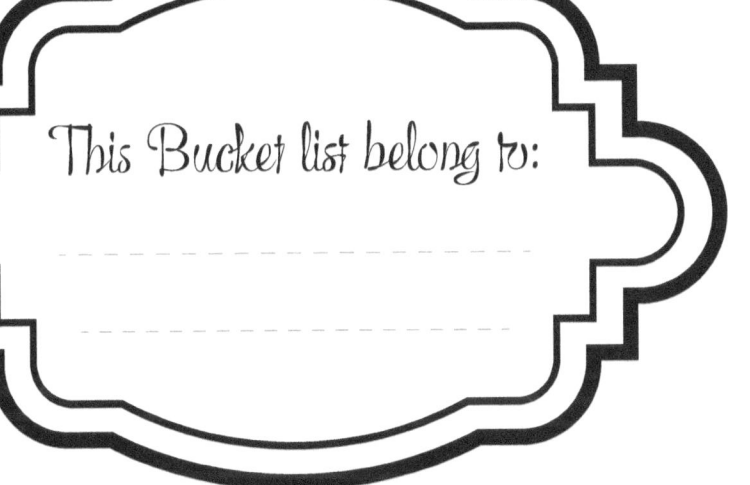

This Bucket list belong to:

_____

_____

# My Bucket List Goal

Date _____ Location _____

Reason of doing this:

_____
_____
_____
_____

Actions we have to take:

_____
_____
_____
_____
_____
_____

My Experience:

_____
_____
_____
_____
_____

# My Bucket List Goal

Date _____ Location _____

Reason of doing this:

_____

_____

_____

_____

Actions we have to take:

_____

_____

_____

_____

_____

My Experience:

_____

_____

_____

_____

# My Bucket List Goal _____
_____

Date _____ Location _____

Reason of doing this:

------------------------------------------------
------------------------------------------------
------------------------------------------------
------------------------------------------------

Actions we have to take:

------------------------------------------------
------------------------------------------------
------------------------------------------------
------------------------------------------------
------------------------------------------------
------------------------------------------------

My Experience:

------------------------------------------------
------------------------------------------------
------------------------------------------------
------------------------------------------------
------------------------------------------------
------------------------------------------------

# My Bucket List Goal _____

_____

Date _____ Location _____

Reason of doing this:

_____

_____

_____

_____


Actions we have to take:

_____

_____

_____

_____

_____


My Experience:

_____

_____

_____

_____

_____

_____

# My Bucket List Goal

Date _____ Location _____

Reason of doing this:

Actions we have to take:

My Experience:

# My Bucket List Goal ----------------
----------------------------------------

Date ------------ Location ----------------

Reason of doing this:
--------------------------------------
--------------------------------------
--------------------------------------
--------------------------------------

Actions we have to take:
--------------------------------------
--------------------------------------
--------------------------------------
--------------------------------------
--------------------------------------
--------------------------------------

My Experience:
--------------------------------------
--------------------------------------
--------------------------------------
--------------------------------------
--------------------------------------
--------------------------------------

# My Bucket List Goal

Date _____ Location _____

Reason of doing this:

_____
_____
_____
_____

Actions we have to take:

_____
_____
_____
_____
_____
_____

My Experience:

_____
_____
_____
_____
_____

# My Bucket List Goal

Date _____ Location _____

Reason of doing this:

_____
_____
_____
_____

Actions we have to take:

_____
_____
_____
_____
_____

My Experience:

_____
_____
_____
_____
_____

# My Bucket List Goal _____

_____

Date _____ Location _____

Reason of doing this:

_____
_____
_____
_____

Actions we have to take:

_____
_____
_____
_____
_____
_____

My Experience:

_____
_____
_____
_____
_____
_____

# My Bucket List Goal _____

_____

Date _____    Location _____

Reason of doing this:

----------------------------------------

----------------------------------------

----------------------------------------

----------------------------------------

Actions we have to take:

----------------------------------------

----------------------------------------

----------------------------------------

----------------------------------------

----------------------------------------

----------------------------------------

My Experience:

----------------------------------------

----------------------------------------

----------------------------------------

----------------------------------------

----------------------------------------

----------------------------------------

# My Bucket List Goal _____
_____

Date _____ Location _____

Reason of doing this:

_____
_____
_____
_____

Actions we have to take:

_____
_____
_____
_____
_____
_____

My Experience:

_____
_____
_____
_____
_____

# My Bucket List Goal _____

Date _____ Location _____

Reason of doing this:

_____
_____
_____
_____

Actions we have to take:

_____
_____
_____
_____
_____
_____

My Experience:

_____
_____
_____
_____
_____

# My Bucket List Goal

Date _____     Location _____

Reason of doing this:

_____

_____

_____

_____

Actions we have to take:

_____

_____

_____

_____

_____

My Experience:

_____

_____

_____

_____

_____

# My Bucket List Goal

Date _____ Location _____

Reason of doing this:

_____

_____

_____

_____

Actions we have to take:

_____

_____

_____

_____

_____

_____

My Experience:

_____

_____

_____

_____

# My Bucket List Goal _____

_____

Date _____ Location _____

Reason of doing this:

_____
_____
_____
_____

Actions we have to take:

_____
_____
_____
_____
_____
_____

My Experience:

_____
_____
_____
_____
_____
_____

# My Bucket List Goal

Date _____    Location _____

Reason of doing this:

_____
_____
_____
_____

Actions we have to take:

_____
_____
_____
_____
_____
_____

My Experience:

_____
_____
_____
_____
_____
_____

# My Bucket List Goal

Date ............................ Location ....................................

Reason of doing this:

.................................................................................

.................................................................................

.................................................................................

.................................................................................

Actions we have to take:

.................................................................................

.................................................................................

.................................................................................

.................................................................................

.................................................................................

.................................................................................

My Experience:

.................................................................................

.................................................................................

.................................................................................

.................................................................................

.................................................................................

# My Bucket List Goal

Date _____ Location _____

Reason of doing this:

_____
_____
_____
_____

Actions we have to take:

_____
_____
_____
_____
_____
_____

My Experience:

_____
_____
_____
_____
_____

# My Bucket List Goal

_____

_____

Date _____ Location _____

Reason of doing this:

_____

_____

_____

_____

Actions we have to take:

_____

_____

_____

_____

_____

My Experience:

_____

_____

_____

_____

_____

# My Bucket List Goal

Date _____ Location _____

Reason of doing this:

_____
_____
_____
_____

Actions we have to take:

_____
_____
_____
_____
_____
_____

My Experience:

_____
_____
_____
_____

# My Bucket List Goal _____

_____

Date _____  Location _____

Reason of doing this:

_____
_____
_____
_____

Actions we have to take:

_____
_____
_____
_____
_____
_____

My Experience:

_____
_____
_____
_____
_____
_____

# My Bucket List Goal ........

Date ............ Location ............

Reason of doing this:

--------------------------------
--------------------------------
--------------------------------
--------------------------------

Actions we have to take:

--------------------------------
--------------------------------
--------------------------------
--------------------------------
--------------------------------

My Experience:

--------------------------------
--------------------------------
--------------------------------
--------------------------------
--------------------------------
--------------------------------

# My Bucket List Goal _____

_____

Date _____ Location _____

Reason of doing this:

_____

_____

_____

_____

Actions we have to take:

_____

_____

_____

_____

_____

_____

My Experience:

_____

_____

_____

_____

_____

_____

# My Bucket List Goal _____

_____

Date _____ Location _____

Reason of doing this:

_____
_____
_____
_____

Actions we have to take:

_____
_____
_____
_____
_____
_____

My Experience:

_____
_____
_____
_____
_____
_____

# My Bucket List Goal

Date _____ Location _____

Reason of doing this:

_____

_____

_____

_____

Actions we have to take:

_____

_____

_____

_____

_____

My Experience:

_____

_____

_____

_____

_____

# My Bucket List Goal

Date _____ Location _____

Reason of doing this:

_____
_____
_____
_____

Actions we have to take:

_____
_____
_____
_____
_____

My Experience:

_____
_____
_____
_____
_____

# My Bucket List Goal

_____

_____

Date _____ Location _____

Reason of doing this:

_____

_____

_____

_____

Actions we have to take:

_____

_____

_____

_____

_____

My Experience:

_____

_____

_____

_____

_____

# My Bucket List Goal

Date _____ Location _____

Reason of doing this:

_____

_____

_____

_____

Actions we have to take:

_____

_____

_____

_____

_____

_____

My Experience:

_____

_____

_____

_____

_____

_____

# My Bucket List Goal _____

_____

Date _____ Location _____

Reason of doing this:
_____
_____
_____
_____

Actions we have to take:
_____
_____
_____
_____
_____

My Experience:
_____
_____
_____
_____
_____

# My Bucket List Goal

Date _____ Location _____

Reason of doing this:

_____
_____
_____
_____

Actions we have to take:

_____
_____
_____
_____
_____
_____

My Experience:

_____
_____
_____
_____
_____
_____

# My Bucket List Goal ......................................................................

........................................................................................................

Date ............................. Location ...........................................

Reason of doing this:

........................................................................................................

........................................................................................................

........................................................................................................

........................................................................................................

Actions we have to take:

........................................................................................................

........................................................................................................

........................................................................................................

........................................................................................................

........................................................................................................

........................................................................................................

My Experience:

........................................................................................................

........................................................................................................

........................................................................................................

........................................................................................................

........................................................................................................

# My Bucket List Goal

Date _____  Location _____

Reason of doing this:

_____

_____

_____

_____

Actions we have to take:

_____

_____

_____

_____

_____

_____

My Experience:

_____

_____

_____

_____

_____

# My Bucket List Goal

Date _____ Location _____

Reason of doing this:

_____
_____
_____
_____

Actions we have to take:

_____
_____
_____
_____
_____
_____

My Experience:

_____
_____
_____
_____
_____
_____

# My Bucket List Goal

Date _____ Location _____

Reason of doing this:

_____

_____

_____

_____

Actions we have to take:

_____

_____

_____

_____

_____

_____

My Experience:

_____

_____

_____

_____

_____

_____

# My Bucket List Goal

Date _____ Location _____

Reason of doing this:

_____

_____

_____

_____

Actions we have to take:

_____

_____

_____

_____

_____

_____

My Experience:

_____

_____

_____

_____

_____

# My Bucket List Goal _____

Date _____ Location _____

Reason of doing this:

_____
_____
_____
_____

Actions we have to take:

_____
_____
_____
_____
_____
_____

My Experience:

_____
_____
_____
_____
_____
_____

# My Bucket List Goal

Date _____ Location _____

Reason of doing this:

_____

_____

_____

_____

Actions we have to take:

_____

_____

_____

_____

_____

My Experience:

_____

_____

_____

_____

_____

# My Bucket List Goal _____

_____

Date _____ Location _____

Reason of doing this:

------------------------------------------

------------------------------------------

------------------------------------------

------------------------------------------

Actions we have to take:

------------------------------------------

------------------------------------------

------------------------------------------

------------------------------------------

------------------------------------------

My Experience:

------------------------------------------

------------------------------------------

------------------------------------------

------------------------------------------

------------------------------------------

# My Bucket List Goal _____

_____

Date _____ Location _____

Reason of doing this:

- - - - - - - - - - - - - - - - - - - - - - - - - - - - - - - -
- - - - - - - - - - - - - - - - - - - - - - - - - - - - - - - -
- - - - - - - - - - - - - - - - - - - - - - - - - - - - - - - -
- - - - - - - - - - - - - - - - - - - - - - - - - - - - - - - -

Actions we have to take:

- - - - - - - - - - - - - - - - - - - - - - - - - - - - - - - -
- - - - - - - - - - - - - - - - - - - - - - - - - - - - - - - -
- - - - - - - - - - - - - - - - - - - - - - - - - - - - - - - -
- - - - - - - - - - - - - - - - - - - - - - - - - - - - - - - -
- - - - - - - - - - - - - - - - - - - - - - - - - - - - - - - -
- - - - - - - - - - - - - - - - - - - - - - - - - - - - - - - -

My Experience:

- - - - - - - - - - - - - - - - - - - - - - - - - - - - - - - -
- - - - - - - - - - - - - - - - - - - - - - - - - - - - - - - -
- - - - - - - - - - - - - - - - - - - - - - - - - - - - - - - -
- - - - - - - - - - - - - - - - - - - - - - - - - - - - - - - -
- - - - - - - - - - - - - - - - - - - - - - - - - - - - - - - -

# My Bucket List Goal ........................

..................................................

Date ........................ Location ........................

Reason of doing this:

---------------------------------------------

---------------------------------------------

---------------------------------------------

---------------------------------------------

Actions we have to take:

---------------------------------------------

---------------------------------------------

---------------------------------------------

---------------------------------------------

---------------------------------------------

My Experience:

---------------------------------------------

---------------------------------------------

---------------------------------------------

---------------------------------------------

---------------------------------------------

# My Bucket List Goal ........

........

Date ........ Location ........

Reason of doing this:

........

........

........

........

Actions we have to take:

........

........

........

........

........

........

My Experience:

........

........

........

........

........

# My Bucket List Goal _____

Date _____ Location _____

Reason of doing this:
_____
_____
_____
_____

Actions we have to take:
_____
_____
_____
_____
_____

My Experience:
_____
_____
_____
_____
_____
_____

# My Bucket List Goal ....................

Date ................. Location .................

Reason of doing this:

------------------------------------------
------------------------------------------
------------------------------------------
------------------------------------------

Actions we have to take:

------------------------------------------
------------------------------------------
------------------------------------------
------------------------------------------
------------------------------------------

My Experience:

------------------------------------------
------------------------------------------
------------------------------------------
------------------------------------------
------------------------------------------

# My Bucket List Goal _____

_____

Date _____    Location _____

Reason of doing this:

_____
_____
_____
_____

Actions we have to take:

_____
_____
_____
_____
_____
_____

My Experience:

_____
_____
_____
_____
_____
_____

# My Bucket List Goal _____

_____

Date _____ Location _____

Reason of doing this:

_____
_____
_____
_____

Actions we have to take:

_____
_____
_____
_____
_____
_____

My Experience:

_____
_____
_____
_____
_____

# My Bucket List Goal ........

Date ........ Location ........

Reason of doing this:

........
........
........
........

Actions we have to take:

........
........
........
........
........

My Experience:

........
........
........
........
........

# My Bucket List Goal ......................................

.............................................................

Date ....................  Location ....................

Reason of doing this:

-------------------------------------------------------------
-------------------------------------------------------------
-------------------------------------------------------------
-------------------------------------------------------------

Actions we have to take:

-------------------------------------------------------------
-------------------------------------------------------------
-------------------------------------------------------------
-------------------------------------------------------------
-------------------------------------------------------------
-------------------------------------------------------------

My Experience:

-------------------------------------------------------------
-------------------------------------------------------------
-------------------------------------------------------------
-------------------------------------------------------------
-------------------------------------------------------------

# My Bucket List Goal

Date _____ Location _____

Reason of doing this:

_____

_____

_____

_____

Actions we have to take:

_____

_____

_____

_____

_____

_____

My Experience:

_____

_____

_____

_____

_____

_____

# My Bucket List Goal

Date _____ Location _____

Reason of doing this:

_____
_____
_____
_____

Actions we have to take:

_____
_____
_____
_____
_____

My Experience:

_____
_____
_____
_____
_____

# My Bucket List Goal

Date _____ Location _____

Reason of doing this:

_____

_____

_____

_____

Actions we have to take:

_____

_____

_____

_____

_____

_____

My Experience:

_____

_____

_____

_____

_____

# My Bucket List Goal _____

_____

Date _____ Location _____

Reason of doing this:

_____
_____
_____
_____

Actions we have to take:

_____
_____
_____
_____
_____
_____

My Experience:

_____
_____
_____
_____
_____
_____

# My Bucket List Goal _____

Date _____          Location _____

Reason of doing this:

_____

_____

_____

_____

Actions we have to take:

_____

_____

_____

_____

_____

_____

My Experience:

_____

_____

_____

_____

_____

_____

# My Bucket List Goal _____

_____

Date _____    Location _____

Reason of doing this:

_____
_____
_____
_____

Actions we have to take:

_____
_____
_____
_____
_____
_____

My Experience:

_____
_____
_____
_____
_____
_____

# My Bucket List Goal _____

_____

Date _____ Location _____

Reason of doing this:

_____
_____
_____
_____

Actions we have to take:

_____
_____
_____
_____
_____
_____

My Experience:

_____
_____
_____
_____
_____
_____

# My Bucket List Goal _____

_____

Date _____ Location _____

Reason of doing this:

_____
_____
_____
_____

Actions we have to take:

_____
_____
_____
_____
_____
_____

My Experience:

_____
_____
_____
_____
_____
_____

# My Bucket List Goal _____

_____

Date _____     Location _____

Reason of doing this:

- - - - - - - - - - - - - - - - - - - - - - - - - - - - - - - - - - - - - -

- - - - - - - - - - - - - - - - - - - - - - - - - - - - - - - - - - - - - -

- - - - - - - - - - - - - - - - - - - - - - - - - - - - - - - - - - - - - -

- - - - - - - - - - - - - - - - - - - - - - - - - - - - - - - - - - - - - -

Actions we have to take:

- - - - - - - - - - - - - - - - - - - - - - - - - - - - - - - - - - - - - -

- - - - - - - - - - - - - - - - - - - - - - - - - - - - - - - - - - - - - -

- - - - - - - - - - - - - - - - - - - - - - - - - - - - - - - - - - - - - -

- - - - - - - - - - - - - - - - - - - - - - - - - - - - - - - - - - - - - -

- - - - - - - - - - - - - - - - - - - - - - - - - - - - - - - - - - - - - -

- - - - - - - - - - - - - - - - - - - - - - - - - - - - - - - - - - - - - -

My Experience:

- - - - - - - - - - - - - - - - - - - - - - - - - - - - - - - - - - - - - -

- - - - - - - - - - - - - - - - - - - - - - - - - - - - - - - - - - - - - -

- - - - - - - - - - - - - - - - - - - - - - - - - - - - - - - - - - - - - -

- - - - - - - - - - - - - - - - - - - - - - - - - - - - - - - - - - - - - -

- - - - - - - - - - - - - - - - - - - - - - - - - - - - - - - - - - - - - -

- - - - - - - - - - - - - - - - - - - - - - - - - - - - - - - - - - - - - -

# My Bucket List Goal _____

_____

Date _____ Location _____

Reason of doing this:

_____
_____
_____
_____

Actions we have to take:

_____
_____
_____
_____
_____
_____

My Experience:

_____
_____
_____
_____
_____
_____

# My Bucket List Goal _____

Date _____  Location _____

Reason of doing this:

_____
_____
_____
_____

Actions we have to take:

_____
_____
_____
_____
_____
_____

My Experience:

_____
_____
_____
_____
_____
_____

# My Bucket List Goal

Date _____ Location _____

Reason of doing this:

_____

_____

_____

_____

Actions we have to take:

_____

_____

_____

_____

_____

My Experience:

_____

_____

_____

_____

_____

# My Bucket List Goal _____

_____

Date _____ Location _____

Reason of doing this:

_____
_____
_____
_____

Actions we have to take:

_____
_____
_____
_____
_____
_____

My Experience:

_____
_____
_____
_____
_____
_____

# My Bucket List Goal _____

_____

Date _____ Location _____

Reason of doing this:

_____
_____
_____
_____

Actions we have to take:

_____
_____
_____
_____
_____
_____

My Experience:

_____
_____
_____
_____
_____

# My Bucket List Goal

Date _____ Location _____

Reason of doing this:

_____
_____
_____
_____

Actions we have to take:

_____
_____
_____
_____
_____
_____

My Experience:

_____
_____
_____
_____
_____
_____

# My Bucket List Goal _____

Date _____  Location _____

Reason of doing this:
----
----
----
----

Actions we have to take:
----
----
----
----
----

My Experience:
----
----
----
----
----
----

# My Bucket List Goal ........................

Date ................. Location .................

Reason of doing this:

------------------------------------

------------------------------------

------------------------------------

------------------------------------

Actions we have to take:

------------------------------------

------------------------------------

------------------------------------

------------------------------------

------------------------------------

------------------------------------

My Experience:

------------------------------------

------------------------------------

------------------------------------

------------------------------------

------------------------------------

------------------------------------

# My Bucket List Goal _____

_____

Date _____ Location _____

Reason of doing this:

_____

_____

_____

_____

Actions we have to take:

_____

_____

_____

_____

_____

My Experience:

_____

_____

_____

_____

_____

# My Bucket List Goal _____

Date _____ Location _____

Reason of doing this:

_____
_____
_____
_____

Actions we have to take:

_____
_____
_____
_____
_____
_____

My Experience:

_____
_____
_____
_____
_____
_____

# My Bucket List Goal

Date _____ Location _____

Reason of doing this:

_____
_____
_____
_____

Actions we have to take:

_____
_____
_____
_____
_____

My Experience:

_____
_____
_____
_____
_____

# My Bucket List Goal _____

_____

Date _____ Location _____

Reason of doing this:

_____

_____

_____

_____

Actions we have to take:

_____

_____

_____

_____

_____

My Experience:

_____

_____

_____

_____

_____

_____

# My Bucket List Goal _____

_____

Date _____ Location _____

Reason of doing this:

_____

_____

_____

_____

Actions we have to take:

_____

_____

_____

_____

_____

My Experience:

_____

_____

_____

_____

_____

# My Bucket List Goal

Date _____ Location _____

Reason of doing this:
_____
_____
_____
_____

Actions we have to take:
_____
_____
_____
_____
_____
_____

My Experience:
_____
_____
_____
_____
_____
_____

# My Bucket List Goal _____

_____

Date _____ Location _____

Reason of doing this:

_____
_____
_____
_____

Actions we have to take:

_____
_____
_____
_____
_____
_____

My Experience:

_____
_____
_____
_____
_____
_____

# My Bucket List Goal _____

_____

Date _____ Location _____

Reason of doing this:

_____
_____
_____
_____

Actions we have to take:

_____
_____
_____
_____
_____
_____

My Experience:

_____
_____
_____
_____
_____
_____

# My Bucket List Goal

Date _____ Location _____

Reason of doing this:

_____
_____
_____
_____

Actions we have to take:

_____
_____
_____
_____
_____

My Experience:

_____
_____
_____
_____
_____

# My Bucket List Goal

Date _____ Location _____

Reason of doing this:

_____

_____

_____

_____

Actions we have to take:

_____

_____

_____

_____

_____

_____

My Experience:

_____

_____

_____

_____

_____

_____

# My Bucket List Goal

Date _____ Location _____

Reason of doing this:

Actions we have to take:

My Experience:

# My Bucket List Goal

Date _____ Location _____

Reason of doing this:

Actions we have to take:

My Experience:

# My Bucket List Goal

Date _____ Location _____

Reason of doing this:

_____

_____

_____

_____

Actions we have to take:

_____

_____

_____

_____

_____

My Experience:

_____

_____

_____

_____

_____

_____

# My Bucket List Goal _____

Date _____ Location _____

Reason of doing this:

_____

_____

_____

_____

Actions we have to take:

_____

_____

_____

_____

_____

_____

My Experience:

_____

_____

_____

_____

_____

_____

# My Bucket List Goal

Date _____ Location _____

Reason of doing this:

_____
_____
_____
_____

Actions we have to take:

_____
_____
_____
_____
_____
_____

My Experience:

_____
_____
_____
_____
_____

# My Bucket List Goal

Date _____ Location _____

Reason of doing this:

_____
_____
_____
_____

Actions we have to take:

_____
_____
_____
_____
_____

My Experience:

_____
_____
_____
_____
_____
_____

# My Bucket List Goal _____

_____

Date _____ Location _____

Reason of doing this:

_____

_____

_____

_____

Actions we have to take:

_____

_____

_____

_____

_____

_____

My Experience:

_____

_____

_____

_____

_____

# My Bucket List Goal _____

_____

Date _____ Location _____

Reason of doing this:

_____
_____
_____
_____

Actions we have to take:

_____
_____
_____
_____
_____
_____

My Experience:

_____
_____
_____
_____
_____
_____

# My Bucket List Goal _____

_____

Date _____ Location _____

Reason of doing this:

_____

_____

_____

_____

Actions we have to take:

_____

_____

_____

_____

_____

My Experience:

_____

_____

_____

_____

_____

_____

# My Bucket List Goal _____

_____

Date _____    Location _____

Reason of doing this:

_____

_____

_____

_____

Actions we have to take:

_____

_____

_____

_____

_____

_____

My Experience:

_____

_____

_____

_____

_____

_____

# My Bucket List Goal

Date _____ Location _____

Reason of doing this:

_____
_____
_____
_____

Actions we have to take:

_____
_____
_____
_____

My Experience:

_____
_____
_____
_____
_____

# My Bucket List Goal _____

Date _____     Location _____

Reason of doing this:

--------------------------------------------

--------------------------------------------

--------------------------------------------

--------------------------------------------

Actions we have to take:

--------------------------------------------

--------------------------------------------

--------------------------------------------

--------------------------------------------

--------------------------------------------

--------------------------------------------

My Experience:

--------------------------------------------

--------------------------------------------

--------------------------------------------

--------------------------------------------

--------------------------------------------

--------------------------------------------

# My Bucket List Goal ......................
................................................................

Date ................ Location ................

Reason of doing this:
................................................................
................................................................
................................................................
................................................................

Actions we have to take:
................................................................
................................................................
................................................................
................................................................
................................................................

My Experience:
................................................................
................................................................
................................................................
................................................................
................................................................

# My Bucket List Goal

Date _____ Location _____

Reason of doing this:

_____
_____
_____
_____

Actions we have to take:

_____
_____
_____
_____
_____

My Experience:

_____
_____
_____
_____
_____

# My Bucket List Goal

Date _____ Location _____

Reason of doing this:

_____
_____
_____
_____

Actions we have to take:

_____
_____
_____
_____
_____
_____

My Experience:

_____
_____
_____
_____
_____
_____

# My Bucket List Goal _____

_____

Date _____ Location _____

Reason of doing this:

_____

_____

_____

_____

Actions we have to take:

_____

_____

_____

_____

_____

_____

My Experience:

_____

_____

_____

_____

_____

_____

# My Bucket List Goal _____

_____

Date _____ Location _____

Reason of doing this:

_____
_____
_____
_____

Actions we have to take:

_____
_____
_____
_____
_____

My Experience:

_____
_____
_____
_____
_____

# My Bucket List Goal

Date _____ Location _____

Reason of doing this:

_____
_____
_____
_____

Actions we have to take:

_____
_____
_____
_____
_____

My Experience:

_____
_____
_____
_____
_____
_____

# My Bucket List Goal _____

_____

Date _____ Location _____

Reason of doing this:

_____
_____
_____
_____

Actions we have to take:

_____
_____
_____
_____
_____
_____

My Experience:

_____
_____
_____
_____
_____
_____

# My Bucket List Goal _____

_____

Date _____     Location _____

Reason of doing this:

- - - - - - - - - - - - - - - - - - - - - - - - - - - - -

- - - - - - - - - - - - - - - - - - - - - - - - - - - - -

- - - - - - - - - - - - - - - - - - - - - - - - - - - - -

- - - - - - - - - - - - - - - - - - - - - - - - - - - - -

Actions we have to take:

- - - - - - - - - - - - - - - - - - - - - - - - - - - - -

- - - - - - - - - - - - - - - - - - - - - - - - - - - - -

- - - - - - - - - - - - - - - - - - - - - - - - - - - - -

- - - - - - - - - - - - - - - - - - - - - - - - - - - - -

- - - - - - - - - - - - - - - - - - - - - - - - - - - - -

My Experience:

- - - - - - - - - - - - - - - - - - - - - - - - - - - - -

- - - - - - - - - - - - - - - - - - - - - - - - - - - - -

- - - - - - - - - - - - - - - - - - - - - - - - - - - - -

- - - - - - - - - - - - - - - - - - - - - - - - - - - - -

# My Bucket List Goal

Date _____ Location _____

Reason of doing this:

_____
_____
_____
_____

Actions we have to take:

_____
_____
_____
_____
_____

My Experience:

_____
_____
_____
_____
_____

# My Bucket List Goal ........

Date ............ Location ............

Reason of doing this:

.......................................
.......................................
.......................................
.......................................

Actions we have to take:

.......................................
.......................................
.......................................
.......................................
.......................................

My Experience:

.......................................
.......................................
.......................................
.......................................
.......................................

# My Bucket List Goal

_____

_____

Date _____ Location _____

Reason of doing this:

_____

_____

_____

_____

Actions we have to take:

_____

_____

_____

_____

_____

My Experience:

_____

_____

_____

_____

_____

# My Bucket List Goal _____

_____

Date _____ Location _____

Reason of doing this:

_____
_____
_____
_____

Actions we have to take:

_____
_____
_____
_____
_____
_____
_____

My Experience:

_____
_____
_____
_____
_____

# My Bucket List Goal

Date _____ Location _____

Reason of doing this:

_____

_____

_____

_____

Actions we have to take:

_____

_____

_____

_____

_____

_____

My Experience:

_____

_____

_____

_____

_____

_____

# My Bucket List Goal

Date _____ Location _____

Reason of doing this:

_____
_____
_____
_____

Actions we have to take:

_____
_____
_____
_____
_____
_____

My Experience:

_____
_____
_____
_____
_____
_____

# My Bucket List Goal _____

_____

Date _____ Location _____

Reason of doing this:

_____
_____
_____
_____

Actions we have to take:

_____
_____
_____
_____
_____

My Experience:

_____
_____
_____
_____
_____
_____

# My Bucket List Goal _____

_____

Date _____ Location _____

Reason of doing this:
_____
_____
_____
_____

Actions we have to take:
_____
_____
_____
_____
_____
_____

My Experience:
_____
_____
_____
_____
_____
_____

# My Bucket List Goal

Date _____ Location _____

Reason of doing this:

_____
_____
_____
_____

Actions we have to take:

_____
_____
_____
_____
_____
_____

My Experience:

_____
_____
_____
_____
_____
_____

# My Bucket List Goal

Date _____ Location _____

Reason of doing this:

_____
_____
_____
_____

Actions we have to take:

_____
_____
_____
_____
_____
_____

My Experience:

_____
_____
_____
_____
_____

# My Bucket List Goal

........................................

........................................

Date ............... Location ...............

Reason of doing this:

........................................

........................................

........................................

........................................

Actions we have to take:

........................................

........................................

........................................

........................................

........................................

........................................

My Experience:

........................................

........................................

........................................

........................................

........................................

........................................

# My Bucket List Goal

Date _____ Location _____

Reason of doing this:

_____

_____

_____

_____

Actions we have to take:

_____

_____

_____

_____

_____

My Experience:

_____

_____

_____

_____

_____

# My Bucket List Goal ........................

........................................................

Date ............................ Location ..................

Reason of doing this:

........................................................

........................................................

........................................................

........................................................

Actions we have to take:

........................................................

........................................................

........................................................

........................................................

........................................................

........................................................

My Experience:

........................................................

........................................................

........................................................

........................................................

........................................................

# My Bucket List Goal

Date _____     Location _____

Reason of doing this:

_____
_____
_____
_____

Actions we have to take:

_____
_____
_____
_____
_____

My Experience:

_____
_____
_____
_____
_____

www.ingramcontent.com/pod-product-compliance
Lightning Source LLC
Chambersburg PA
CBHW020543220526
45463CB00006B/2174